What Your Body Says

The Secrets of Nonverbal Sexual Communication, Understanding Nonverbal Cues during Sex and the Art of Nonverbal Seduction

Cheryl Bach

What Your Body Says

Cheryl Bach

Table of Contents

What Your Body Says

Cheryl Bach

What Your Body Says

Chapter 1

Introduction

Sexuality is an essential component of human behavior, with the erotic arts and love existing long before technology or culture was present. From the ancient texts to modern media, pleasure, and intimacy is celebrated and shared, while courting and seduction pressing forward. Communication amongst humans has always been excessively nonverbal. So sexual communication has been no exception.

Nonverbal sexual communication refers to the various ways in which individuals express their sexual desires, thoughts, and feelings through bodily signals and cues. The way we react and respond during intimate moments reveals a lot about our sexual preferences, comfort levels, and boundaries. These signals can manifest in various forms, including body language, facial expressions, tone of voice, and physical touch.

Why Knowing the Art of Nonverbal Seduction Is Important

The art of nonverbal seduction plays a significant role in sexual encounters because it allows individuals to communicate their desires, needs, and boundaries without relying solely on verbal communication. Nonverbal cues can make up as much as 90% of our communication, with the remaining 10% being verbal. Therefore, being skilled in the art of nonverbal seduction can help individuals more effectively convey their intentions and better understand their partner's desires during sex.

Moreover, nonverbal communication can also enhance intimacy between partners. Consensual sexual touch is an essential part of promoting healthy relationships, creating trust, and improving mental health. These aspects often lead to mutual physical motivation, including pleasure, as well as responses to sensual stroking, touch, and intercourse.

Understanding Nonverbal Cues during Sex

One of the most critical aspects of nonverbal communication during sex is the ability to read and interpret cues accurately. This includes recognizing signs of pleasure, discomfort, or dissatisfaction in your partner's body language, facial expressions, and tone of voice. By understanding and responding to these cues, individuals can ensure a more satisfying sexual experience for both themselves and their partners.

Additionally, nonverbal communication involves setting boundaries and respecting them. It is essential to pay attention to signals that indicate discomfort or a lack of enthusiasm from your partner. Having open and honest communication about boundaries and consent is crucial for creating a safe and consensual sexual environment while enhancing intimacy and trust between partners.

Finally, mastering the art of nonverbal seduction can add a level of intensity and excitement to sexual encounters. Nonverbal cues such as eye contact, body positioning, and subtle touches can build sexual tension and connection between partners while heightening arousal levels and leading to more pleasurable experiences.

In conclusion, nonverbal sexual communication is an essential part of sexual encounters. It involves nonverbal cues such as body language, facial expressions, and tone of voice to express one's sexual desires effectively, boundaries, and feelings even without verbal communication. Mastering the art of nonverbal seduction can enhance the sexual experience and improve the intimacy and pleasure between partners. Understanding nonverbal cues is crucial for creating a safe and consensual sexual environment, leading to more satisfying sexual interactions. The following chapters in this book will delve into different nonverbal cues and how to interpret them, setting boundaries, and improving communication during sexual encounters.

What Your Body Says

Chapter 2

Body Language during Intimacy

During intimate moments, our bodies can express a vast range of emotions and desires that words cannot always convey. It is important to analyze your body's behavior and understand the different types of body language and their meaning. By paying attention to and interpreting your partner's body language during intimacy, you can enhance your sexual experiences and create a more satisfying and pleasurable encounter.

Understanding Different Types of Body Language

Body language refers to the nonverbal communication conveyed by physical behavior such as posture, gestures, eye contact, facial expressions, and touch. During intimacy, several types of body language can indicate a range of emotions, such as verbal communication, happiness, sadness, anger, or discomfort.

Facial Expressions: Facial expressions are an essential element in nonverbal communication, and they play a vital role in intimacy. Smiling, winking, biting your lips, and eye contact are all examples of how facial expressions can convey feelings of attraction and arousal.

Body Posture: Another critical aspect of body language during intimacy is body posture, such as leaning in or away from your partner. Leaning in can indicate sexual attraction, while leaning away could suggest discomfort or a lack of interest.

Gestures: Touching or caressing one's partner can signify a desire for intimacy, while pushing away or avoiding touch may indicate boundaries or discomfort.

Vocal Cues: Moaning, sighing, and heavy breathing can all be signals of arousal and pleasure, while tense voice and silence could indicate discomfort or dissatisfaction.

How to Interpret Signals from Your Partner

The key to interpreting nonverbal cues during intimacy is to pay close attention to your partner's body language. Look for consistent signals like smiling, eye contact, and touching, which can be signs of attraction and desire.

However, it is also important to look for any subtle changes in your partner's body language that may indicate discomfort or dissatisfaction. These can include avoiding eye contact, tensed muscles, or closed-off body posture.

It is crucial to communicate openly with your partner about what you each like and dislike to ensure a mutually

What Your Body Says

satisfying experience. If you sense any nonverbal cues that suggest discomfort or boundaries, ask your partner if they are comfortable and see if there's anything you can do to make them feel more at ease.

In addition to paying attention to your partner's body language, it's also essential to be aware of your body language and how it may be interpreted by your partner. Consistently looking away, crossing your arms, or avoiding touch can send signals of disinterest or discomfort, making it important to remain open and receptive during intimacy.

How to Enhance Nonverbal Communication during Intimacy

There are several ways to enhance nonverbal communication during intimacy, allowing you and your partner to connect on a deeper and more intimate level.

Cheryl Bach

Firstly, try to maintain eye contact with your partner when connecting physically to show that you're present in the moment and turned on by their attentions. Additionally, use touch to convey your emotions and desires, touching your partner in ways that you find satisfying while reading their reactions.

It is also essential to create a safe environment for open and honest communication during intimacy. By setting boundaries and discussing each other's preferences beforehand, you can enter the experience without fear of misunderstandings or unwanted actions.

Lastly, practice active listening, where both parties can communicate openly and respond to one another's nonverbal cues. This makes the experience enjoyable and intimate for both partners.

What Your Body Says

In Conclusion, nonverbal communication plays a crucial role in creating intimacy and building desire between partners during sex. Understanding different types of body language, paying attention to subtle changes, and interpreting signals from your partner can add depth and connection to intimate moments and sexual experiences. By enhancing nonverbal communication during intimacy, partners can create a safe and pleasurable environment where they can openly communicate their emotions and desires, leading to a deeper and more satisfying sexual experience.

Chapter 3

The Power of Nonverbal Communication in Seduction

Nonverbal communication plays an essential role in seduction, as most relationships are formed through nonverbal communication rather than verbal communication. Nonverbal cues like body posture, gestures, and eye contact can mask countless emotions, and mastering these nonverbal cues can improve your seduction skills drastically.

What Your Body Says

Step-By-Step Guide on How to Communicate through Body Language during Sex

Eye Contact: The eyes are windows to the soul and can be used to convey deep emotions and attraction. Maintaining eye contact while talking or caressing can help you connect with your partner on a more profound level, sending signals of desire and attraction.

Physical Touch: Touch is also a crucial aspect of body language during seduction. Touching another person's hand, shoulders, knees, and other erogenous zones can send signals of attraction and interest. Try to vary your touches: caress, squeeze, nibble, use different pressures and see how your partner reacts.

Facial Expressions: Facial expressions can speak volumes when it comes to seduction. Smiling, biting your lips, and sultry glances are all great ways to indicate attraction and desire.

Body Posture: Your body posture can also signal your intentions during seduction. Leaning toward a person can convey interest, while crossing your arms or turning away can indicate disinterest or discomfort.

Vocal Cues: The way you say things can be more important than what you say. Moaning, sighing, heavy breathing, and subtle verbal cues such as whispers breathlessly into their ear can all set the tone for a seductive encounter.

Techniques to Improve Nonverbal Communication Skills

Practice Active Listening: By actively listening to your partner's nonverbal cues, you can become more attuned to their desires and needs, making it easier to communicate through body language during sex.

What Your Body Says

Develop Self-Awareness: Being self-aware of your body language and how others perceive you is essential in nonverbal communication. Pay attention to your gestures, voice tone, and facial expressions, and work on improving them where necessary.

Learn to Read Nonverbal Cues: Understanding nonverbal cues during seduction is essential. Paying attention to your partner's body language, facial expressions, and vocal cues can help you determine what they want and how to respond.

Mimic Your Partner: Mimicking the physical movements and gestures of your partner during sex can create a deeper sense of connection and understanding, leading to a more satisfying experience for both partners.

Practice Empathy: To effectively communicate through nonverbal cues during sex, you must be empathetic and receptive to your partner's needs. Practicing empathy will help you to understand what your partner desires, leading to better communication and a more satisfying and intimate experience.

Understanding the Difference between Positive and Negative Nonverbal Signals during Seduction

Positive nonverbal signals during seduction include smiling, eye contact, leaning in, touching, and open body language. These signals indicate that your partner is interested and attracted to you.

On the other hand, negative nonverbal cues may include crossing arms, avoiding eye contact, maintaining physical distance, and turning away. These signals suggest a lack of interest or discomfort.

It is important to be attentive to both positive and negative nonverbal signals during seduction and adjust your approach accordingly. If you notice your partner exhibiting negative cues, take a step back and assess the situation before continuing. It is crucial to understand and respect your partner's boundaries and desires to maintain a healthy and respectful relationship.

In conclusion, nonverbal communication is an essential aspect of seduction and can greatly improve the intimacy and connection between partners during sex. By paying attention to nonverbal cues, practicing active listening and empathy, and improving our own body language, we can become better communicators and lovers, leading to deeper and more satisfying sexual experiences for both partners.

Chapter 4

Tips for Improving Nonverbal Communication

Effective nonverbal communication is a crucial aspect of sexual communication that can make or break an intimate experience. Understanding nonverbal cues and how to communicate with them can take your sexual encounters from average to unforgettable. Here are some practical tips for improving nonverbal communication during sex:

Enhancing your Self-Awareness: Body Posture, Eye Contact, etc.

Enhancing self-awareness is the first step in improving nonverbal communication during sex. It involves

What Your Body Says

understanding your own body language, facial expressions, and vocal cues and knowing how you are perceived by your partner.

Paying attention to your posture, maintaining comfortable eye contact, and avoiding nervous gestures, such as fidgeting or playing with your hair, can all signal confidence and interest in your partner.

Importance of Physical Touch and Gestures during Sex

Physical touch and gestures can speak volumes during sex. They can communicate your desires, show gratitude for your partner's actions, and express pleasure or discomfort. When used effectively, they can enhance the sexual experience and lead to a deeper emotional connection.

For example, caressing your partner's face or neck can convey intimacy and tenderness, while grabbing their hair or pulling them closer can signal passion and dominance. When engaging in sexual activity, take every opportunity to use physical touch and gestures to communicate your desires and needs to your partner.

Practicing Mindfulness and Role-playing Exercises to Improve Communication

Practicing mindfulness is a powerful tool for improving nonverbal communication skills in the bedroom. It involves being present in the moment and paying attention to your body, emotions, and sensations. By practicing mindfulness, you can reduce stress and anxiety during sexual encounters, allowing you to communicate more effectively with your partner.

Role-playing exercises can also be an effective way to improve nonverbal communication during sex. These exercises involve taking turns playing different roles and using body language to communicate your desires and needs. For example, one partner can play the submissive role while blindfolded, while the other partner gives them nonverbal commands to follow with body language.

These exercises can build trust and intimacy between partners and improve communication skills outside of the bedroom as well. They can also help to develop a deeper understanding of your partner's body language and nonverbal cues.

In conclusion, effective nonverbal communication during sex can significantly enhance the intimacy and satisfaction experienced by both partners, leading to more fulfilling sexual experiences. By focusing on enhancing self-awareness, physical touch and gestures, practicing mindfulness, and engaging in role-playing exercises to improve communication, you can improve nonverbal communication skills and elevate the sexual experience to new heights.

Remember, nonverbal communication is not a one-size-fits-all approach and can vary depending on cultural background, personality, and relationship history. Therefore, it's essential to pay attention to verbal and nonverbal cues and feedback from your partner to build a deeper connection and ultimately improve sexual satisfaction.

Most importantly, always prioritize open and honest communication with your partner. Verbal communication is just as important as nonverbal communication and can help establish boundaries, desires, and consent. By incorporating both verbal and nonverbal communication, you can bring more awareness to the subtle nuances of your sexual interactions and create a more satisfying and fulfilling experience.

What Your Body Says

With these tips and techniques, you can unlock the art of nonverbal seduction and take your intimacy with your partner to the next level.

Chapter 5

Understanding Nonverbal Signals in Different Stages of Intimacy

Effective communication during sexual interactions is a vital component of an intimate relationship. While verbal communication can be advantageous, nonverbal communication also plays a significant role in sexual encounters, especially during different stages of intimacy. Understanding nonverbal signals can help maintain the momentum and intensity experienced during sex. Here are some tips for understanding nonverbal signals during foreplay, peak excitement, and post-coital moments.

What Your Body Says

Communication during Foreplay

Before you get into the heat of the moment, nonverbal cues can set the tone for the rest of the experience. During foreplay, partners can use nonverbal signals to express interest, attraction, and desire.

Eye contact and maintaining close proximity to your partner's body can signal your interest. Touching your partner's arm or hand can communicate intimacy, while running your fingers through their hair can speak of sensuality.

Body language, such as leaning in towards your partner, can indicate interest. You can also read these signs from your partner's behavior. For example, if they reciprocate your touch or lean in towards you, it is likely that they are interested in continuing the sexual encounter.

Cheryl Bach

It's also important to listen to your own physical responses during foreplay. Are you breathing heavily? Is your heart rate increasing? By recognizing and acknowledging these nonverbal cues, you can better tune into your own desires and communicate them to your partner.

Communication during Peak of Excitement

During the peak of excitement, nonverbal communication becomes even more critical. At this point, partners may become more physically expressive and use nonverbal signals to guide each other.

Moans, groans, and heavy breathing can indicate pleasure and arousal. Vocalizations, particularly in the form of short and sharp breaths, can signal to your partner that they are doing something right. Touching, hugging, and kissing, become more intense during the peak of excitement and can reflect passion and desire.

What Your Body Says

When partners' bodies are moving rhythmically together, there is nonverbal communication being exchanged. The pace and intensity of movement can indicate the level of intensity and satisfaction during sex. Maintaining eye contact can also intensify the sexual experience as it creates a level of intimacy between the partners.

You can use nonverbal communication during the peak of excitement to express desire for certain positions or actions. For example, moving towards your partner's ear and whispering, "I want you to touch me here" can indicate what feels good and what you want your partner to do next.

Communication during Post-Coital Moments

Nonverbal communication during post-coital moments can vary between partners. Some may feel the need to cuddle, while others may prefer to maintain their distance.

Cheryl Bach

Understanding your partner's nonverbal cues during this time is essential to create a harmonious experience.

Cuddling and hugging after sex indicates a desire for intimacy, while reluctance to engage in physical affection can indicate a need for space. A natural inclination towards holding hands or touching each other's hair or face can indicate a deeper emotional connection.

Additionally, facial expressions, including smiling, laughing, or sighing, can communicate feelings of satisfaction and contentment. It's essential to observe what your partner does to understand how they feel and adjust your behavior accordingly.

However, it is important to remember that nonverbal communication during post-coital moments can be complex and vary from person to person. While some partners may want to talk about the experience, others may prefer to stay silent. Paying attention to your partner's body language and facial expressions is essential to learn what they are experiencing.

Nonverbal cues during post-coital moments can also indicate the need for emotional support. For instance, if your partner seems distant or sad, you can initiate a gentle touch or an affectionate hug. This nonverbal communication can convey your empathy and care.

In conclusion, nonverbal communication plays an integral role in sexual encounters as it enhances intimacy, develops trust, and ultimately connects partners on a deeper level. Understanding nonverbal signals during foreplay, peak excitement, and post-coital moments can help increase pleasure, satisfaction, and profound emotional connections. Therefore, it is essential to be mindful of your partner's nonverbal communication and respond appropriately to create a more fulfilling and satisfying sexual experience for both partners.

Remember to listen to your body and communicate your needs and desires in a nonverbal manner, and to read your partner's nonverbal cues to enhance the sexual experience. Communication during sex isn't just about words, but also involves a lot of physicality, connectivity, and emotional connections. Always appreciate and acknowledge your partner's nonverbal signals and work together to create an environment in which you both feel comfortable expressing yourselves authentically.

What Your Body Says

Chapter 6

The Art of Nonverbal Seduction

What is seduction? In its simplest definition, it is the act of persuading someone to do something that they may not have been inclined to do otherwise. When it comes to sexual relationships, seduction is about creating an atmosphere that allows both partners to feel comfortable and open while creating a desire for intimacy.

The Art of Nonverbal Seduction is about using nonverbal cues to communicate your desires and intensify the connection between you and your partner. By mastering this art, you can turn your partner on during foreplay, communicate desire and passion, and create an experience that neither of you will forget.

What Your Body Says

Seduction is both an art and a science. It requires skill, strategy, patience, and a good dose of confidence. While verbal communication plays a vital role in creating sexual tension between partners, nonverbal communication can be even more important when it comes to seduction. The right nonverbal cues can be incredibly powerful, and can make all the difference in turning your partner on and creating a truly intimate and passionate experience.

Mastering the Art of Seduction through Nonverbal Cues

The first step in mastering nonverbal seduction is to understand the power of body language. The way you move, the way you touch, and even the expression on your face can all send powerful messages to your partner. It's important to be aware of your own body language and how it's being received by your partner.

Techniques to Turn Your Partner on During Foreplay Using Nonverbal Signals

Foreplay is an essential part of any sexual encounter, and nonverbal communication plays a crucial role in setting the mood and getting your partner in the right frame of mind. Here are some techniques to turn your partner on using nonverbal signals during foreplay:

Eye Contact: Maintaining eye contact is a powerful nonverbal tool that can communicate deep feelings of intimacy and desire. By locking eyes with your partner, you can build instant attraction and heighten sexual tension.

Touch: Nonverbal touch, such as gentle strokes or caresses, can send shivers down your partner's spine. Use touch to explore your partner's body, paying attention to what areas make them feel most aroused.

What Your Body Says

Body Language: Your body language can speak volumes about your intentions and desires. Lean in close to your partner, tilt your head slightly to the side, and maintain an open posture to show them that you're interested and invested in the moment.

Whisper: Whispering can be an incredibly effective tool in nonverbal seduction as it can create intimacy and build anticipation. Whisper sweet nothings or dirty talk in your partner's ear, and they'll be putty in your hands.

Smiling: A playful smile can be alluring and instantly draw your partner in. Smiling conveys a relaxed and happy demeanor, allowing them to feel safe and secure during the foreplay.

Mirroring: Mirroring is a powerful technique where you match your partner's body language. For example, if they lean in closer, you also lean in. By mirroring their actions, it can make them feel heard, validated and in tune with your desires.

Communicating Desire and Passion through Body Language

Your body language can communicate your internal emotions and desires, even when you're not actively speaking. Here are some tips for communicating desire and passion through body language:

Posture: Stand tall and proud, with your shoulders back and head held high. This communicates confidence and a sense of assertiveness, two qualities that are often associated with sexual attraction.

Facial Expressions: Your facial expressions can communicate everything from joy to lust to intense passion.

What Your Body Says

Make eye contact with your partner, smile, and express your emotions using facial expressions.

Touch: Touch is one of the most powerful tools in nonverbal communication. Caressing, massaging or even gently running your fingers over your partner's skin can communicate desire and arouse them.

Movement: Movement can also be a powerful tool for communication during sex. Whether it's a slow, seductive dance or guiding your partner's hands over your body, movement can communicate passion and desire.

How to Communicate Desire and Passion through Body Language

One way to communicate desire and passion through body language is to use your hips. A simple movement of your hips during sex can convey a sense of wild abandon and intense passion. You could also use your mouth to communicate passion by kissing your partner deeply and passionately.

Another technique is to use your hands to explore your partner's body. Run your fingers over their skin and explore every inch of their body, focusing on the areas that you know will turn them on. This communicates your desire to please them and shows them that you are fully invested in the experience.

You can also use your body language to communicate your excitement and pleasure during sex. Moaning, breathing heavily, and using facial expressions to show your pleasure are all ways to communicate your enthusiasm for what's happening.

In addition to using nonverbal cues to communicate your desire and passion, it's important to pay attention to your partner's nonverbal cues as well. This can help you understand what they like and what they don't like, so that you can better tailor your actions to their desires.

Overall, mastering the art of nonverbal seduction takes practice, patience, and a willingness to be vulnerable with your partner. With the right techniques and a bit of confidence, however, you can create truly intimate and passionate experiences that neither of you will forget. Remember, nonverbal communication is just as important as verbal communication, so take your time to explore what works best for both you and your partner.

Chapter 7

Pitfalls to Avoid in Nonverbal Communication

Nonverbal communication plays an essential role in creating a memorable and intimate sexual experience. However, despite its importance, there are several pitfalls that you need to be aware of to make sure that you're not misreading or sending confusing signals. Below are some common mistakes to avoid while engaging in nonverbal communication.

Misreading Signals

One of the most significant pitfalls in nonverbal communication is misreading signals. It can cause confusion and lead to a negative sexual experience. False interpretations can be quite common if you and your partner are not paying full attention or aren't familiar with each other's nonverbal cues.

To avoid misreading signals, it's important to pay close attention to your partner's body language and make sure you understand their nonverbal cues. Also, it's critical to ask clarifying questions if you're unsure about a particular action or signal. Don't be afraid to speak up and ask what your partner means, as it can prevent misunderstandings and enhance your overall experience.

Cultural Differences in Nonverbal Communication

Cultural differences can also impact nonverbal communication during sex. Gestures or behaviors that are considered acceptable or arousing in one culture may not be viewed the same way in another culture. It is important to keep in mind that our upbringing and cultural experiences can shape our nonverbal expressions of sexuality.

To avoid this pitfall, discuss with your partner what nonverbal cues and behaviors are acceptable to both of you. While it's important to respect each other's cultural backgrounds, it's also essential to establish a mutual understanding of what signals and expressions you'll be using during sex.

How to Avoid Giving Mixed Signals

Mixed signals can occur when your body language and verbal communication don't match up. For instance, saying "no" while at the same time giving off signals that say "yes," or vice versa. Giving mixed signals can lead to confusion, frustration, or can even be harmful in some circumstances.

What Your Body Says

To avoid sending mixed signals, make sure you're aware of how your verbal and nonverbal communication aligns. If you're unsure about sending mixed signals, don't be afraid to communicate with your partner directly and verbally.

Common Mistakes While Reading Body Language

It is essential to note that nonverbal communication is not foolproof and can be misread at times. Some common mistakes that people make while reading body language include relying too heavily on stereotypes, making assumptions without understanding context, or being too quick to draw conclusions.

To avoid these mistakes, it's important to focus on the individual and their specific nonverbal cues, rather than relying on preconceived notions or assumptions. Additionally, take the time to observe the context in which nonverbal communication is occurring as it can provide valuable context clues.

In conclusion, nonverbal communication can play a vital role in creating a memorable and intimate sexual experience. Understanding and avoiding pitfalls in nonverbal communication is essential to ensure that both you and your partner can communicate effectively. By paying close attention to each other's nonverbal cues, respecting cultural differences, avoiding mixed signals, and taking care not to make assumptions, you can enhance your sexual connection and create a more satisfying experience overall.

If you're new to nonverbal communication, take the time to learn about your partner's body language and try different techniques to see what works best for both of you. Remember, nonverbal communication is just as important as verbal communication, so put in the time and effort to hone your skills and improve your intimacy.

What Your Body Says

Overall, by being mindful of the potential pitfalls and working to avoid them, you can master the art of nonverbal communication and create an incredibly intimate and passionate sexual experience for both you and your partner.

Chapter 8

Final Thoughts

Decoding and understanding nonverbal sexual communication is an essential skill for anyone who wants to experience more pleasure, intimacy, and connection during sex. In this book, we explored the art of nonverbal seduction, including understanding the power of eye contact, body language, and the importance of engaging all of your senses.

Benefits of Learning and Mastering Nonverbal Sexual Communication

Learning and mastering nonverbal sexual communication has many benefits. Firstly, it can create a deeper connection with your partner and lead to more satisfying sexual experiences. Nonverbal communication can help you understand what your partner wants or needs, which can lead to greater pleasure and intimacy during sex.

Secondly, mastering nonverbal communication can help you build confidence in your sexual abilities, which can enhance your overall sexual experience. Being able to read and respond to your partner's nonverbal cues can give you a better sense of control during sex, which can help you feel more comfortable trying new things and taking risks.

Finally, mastering nonverbal communication during sex can also help improve your overall communication skills with your partner outside the bedroom. Good communication is vital to the health of any relationship, and understanding nonverbal cues during sex can help you build better communication skills overall.

Importance of Practice and Consistency in Improving Nonverbal Communication Skills

It's important to understand that mastering nonverbal sexual communication takes practice and consistency. It's not something that can be learned overnight, and it takes time and effort to become proficient.

To improve your nonverbal communication skills in bed, it's essential to practice and experiment with different techniques and strategies. You can start by paying more attention to your partner's nonverbal cues during sex and trying to respond to them in a way that amplifies the connection between you two.

Additionally, developing your nonverbal communication skills requires consistency. It's not enough to use these skills every once in a while - you need to make it a regular part of your sexual experience. Consistency will help you develop a strong foundation of nonverbal communication

What Your Body Says

that you can rely on to enhance your sexual connection over time.

Conclusion and Overall Impact of Nonverbal Communication during Sex

In conclusion, mastering nonverbal sexual communication is an essential component of a healthy, satisfying sexual relationship. Understanding the art of nonverbal seduction can help you deepen your connection with your partner, enhance your overall sexual experience and promote better communication skills outside of the bedroom.

By learning how to read and respond to nonverbal cues, you can better understand your partner's desires and needs, leading to a more fulfilling sexual encounter. Consistency in practicing and developing these skills is key to becoming proficient and reaping the benefits of nonverbal communication during sex.

Overall, nonverbal communication is a powerful tool for building deeper and more intimate connections with your partner. When used effectively, it can make your sexual encounters more enjoyable, satisfying, and emotionally fulfilling. Take the time to learn about your partner's body language, experiment with different techniques and make nonverbal communication a regular part of your sexual experience to reap the full benefits of this powerful tool.

What Your Body Says